The Menopause Kitchen:

Natural Foods, Herbs, and Remedies for Hormonal Health

Marigold Ravenwood

Edited by

Dr Magali Chohan

Aromates.clouds.

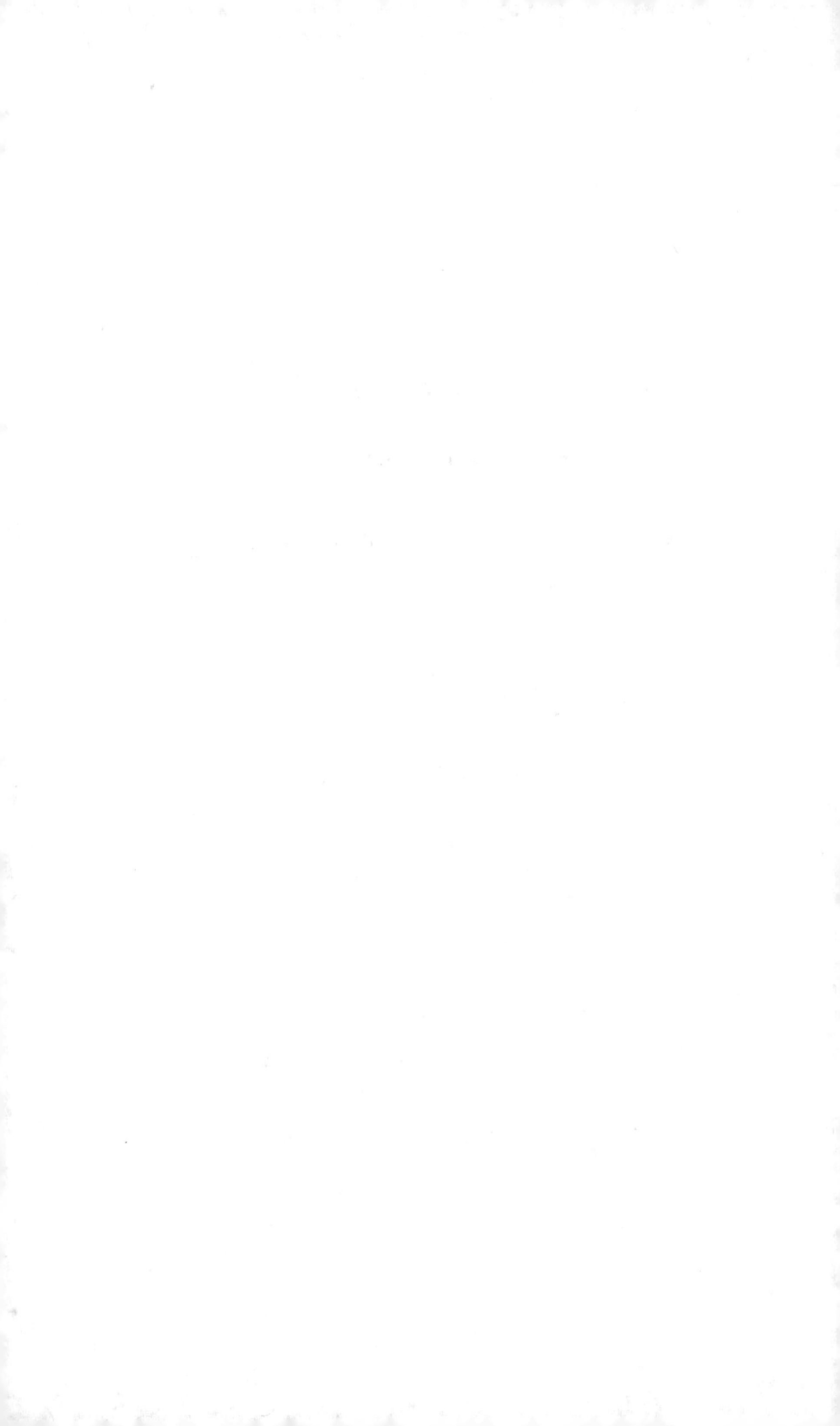

Table of Contents

9 Phytoestrogenic Foods 52

13 Herbals & Nutraceuticals..................106

14 Bibliography.....................................113

1 What is Menopause?

Menopause is a natural biological process that marks the permanent end of menstruation and reproductive capacity in women. It occurs when the ovaries stop producing eggs and there is a decline in the production of hormones like oestrogen and progesterone. Menopause is officially diagnosed after 12 consecutive months without a menstrual period and typically occurs between the ages of 45 and 55, though it can happen earlier or later.

Stages of Menopause

Perimenopause (the transition phase):

- This phase can start several years before menopause as oestrogen levels begin to fluctuate.
- Women may experience irregular periods and symptoms like hot flushes, mood changes, and sleep disturbances.

Menopause:

- o The point at which a woman has not had a period for 12 consecutive months.
- o Ovarian hormone production decreases significantly during this time.

Post menopause:

- o The years after menopause.
- o Symptoms like hot flushes may subside, but the decrease in oestrogen can lead to long-term effects like increased risks of osteoporosis and cardiovascular disease.

Symptoms of Menopause

The experience varies between individuals, but common symptoms include:
- Hot flushes and night sweats
- Mood swings or irritability
- Fatigue and sleep disturbances

- Weight gain or slowed metabolism
- Vaginal dryness
- Reduced libido
- Memory and concentration issues ("brain fog")
- Hair thinning or dryness of skin

Why Does It Happen?

Menopause is a normal part of aging and occurs because the ovaries gradually lose their ability to release eggs and produce reproductive hormones. This hormonal shift affects many systems in the body, causing the associated symptoms.

Premature and Early Menopause

- **Premature menopause:** Occurs before age 40.
- **Early menopause:** Happens between 40 and 45. Both can be caused by genetics, medical treatments like chemotherapy, or surgical removal of the ovaries.

Management and Support

Although menopause is a natural process, its symptoms can impact quality of life. Management strategies include:

- **Lifestyle changes**: Regular exercise, balanced diet, and stress management.
- **Hormone Replacement Therapy (HRT)**: Replaces lost hormones to relieve symptoms.
- **Natural remedies**: Phytoestrogen-rich foods and herbal supplements.
- **Supportive therapies**: Cognitive behavioural therapy, mindfulness, or counselling.

Menopause is a transformative phase, and with the right support and lifestyle adjustments, many women find it an opportunity to focus on their health and well-being.

2 General Nutrition Guidance

Hydration and nutrition can have a significant impact on wellbeing.

Dietary and drinks guidelines[1]:
- Eating at least 5 portions of fruits and vegetables per day (1 portion equals to 80g of fresh, canned, or frosen fruit and vegetables)
- Drinking at least 6-8 glasses of fluids per day (water, low-fat & low-sugar drinks, up to 150mL fruit juices, tea)
- keeping caffeine (tea & coffee) intake down to 2 per day (try decaf in craving)
- Consuming less than 14 units of alcohol per week[2] (6 glasses of wine or 6 pints of beer)

[1] England, P. H. (2016). The Eatwell Guide. Available at: www.gov.uk/government/publications/the-eatwell-guide.

[2] Department of Health (2016) Alcohol Guidelines Review— Report From the Guidelines Development Group to the UK Chief Medical Officers.

3 Menopause Nutrition & Phytoestrogens

For menopausal women in the UK, recent research suggests that a balanced diet rich in phytoestrogens, healthy fats, and proteins, while also moderating carbohydrate intake, can help manage menopausal symptoms and reduce risks for chronic conditions such as heart disease and osteoporosis.

The optimal macronutrient breakdown tends to reflect these priorities [1]

1. **Protein** (25-30% of total calories): Protein plays a key role in preserving muscle mass, which naturally declines during menopause. It is also essential for hormone production and immune function. Sources include lean meats, fish, eggs, legumes, and plant-based options like tofu.

2. **Healthy Fats** (30-35% of total calories): Emphasizing sources like olive oil,

avocado, nuts, and seeds supports hormonal balance, reduces inflammation, and promotes heart health. Omega-3 fatty acids are beneficial for mood regulation and bone health.

3. **Carbohydrates** (35-40% of total calories): Complex carbs like whole grains, vegetables, and fruits are recommended, as they provide steady energy, aid digestion, and help regulate blood sugar. Fiber-rich foods also support gut health, which is often impacted during menopause.

4. **Phytoestrogen-Rich Foods**: A diet rich in soy products, flaxseeds, and other phytoestrogen-rich foods can help balance declining oestrogen levels and alleviate hot flashes and other menopausal symptoms. These can be considered within the carbohydrate and fat percentages.

[1] Silva TR, Oppermann K, Reis FM, Spritzer PM. Nutrition in Menopausal Women: A Narrative Review. *Nutrients.* 2021; 13(7):2149. https://doi.org/10.3390/nu13072149

Phytoestrogens are naturally occurring plant compounds that have a chemical structure similar to oestrogen, the hormone that decreases during menopause. They are known for their ability to mimic or modulate the effects of oestrogen in the body. Here's how they relate to menopause:

How Phytoestrogens Work

Oestrogen-like Activity

Phytoestrogens bind to oestrogen receptors in the body, especially when natural oestrogen levels are low (e.g., during menopause). However, their effects are much weaker compared to the body's natural oestrogen.

Dual Action

Depending on the body's hormonal state, phytoestrogens can either mimic oestrogen when levels are low or block stronger oestrogen activity (as seen in premenopausal women). This makes them selective oestrogen receptor modulators (*SERMs*).

Role in Menopause

Relief from Vasomotor Symptoms

During menopause, hot flushes and night sweats, collectively known as vasomotor symptoms, are common due to hormonal fluctuations. Phytoestrogens, particularly soy isoflavones, mimic oestrogen's effects and have been shown to alleviate the frequency and severity of these symptoms in some women. Regular consumption of phytoestrogen-rich foods or supplements may offer mild to moderate relief over time.

Bone Health

Oestrogen plays a critical role in maintaining bone density by regulating bone remodelling and preserving collagen within the bone matrix. During menopause, declining oestrogen accelerates bone loss, increasing the risk of osteoporosis. Phytoestrogens, especially those from soy and flaxseed, can mimic oestrogenic activity, stimulating osteoblasts (bone-forming cells), slowing bone resorption, and reducing the risk of fractures. Studies suggest that regular intake of phytoestrogen-rich foods or supplements can help protect postmenopausal women against osteoporosis.

Heart Health

Postmenopausal women experience a higher risk of cardiovascular disease, partially due to declining oestrogen, which normally helps maintain healthy cholesterol levels and arterial flexibility. Phytoestrogens, particularly soy isoflavones, have been shown to reduce LDL (bad cholesterol) and increase HDL (good cholesterol), improving overall lipid profiles. Additionally, they may help relax blood vessels and enhance arterial health, reducing the risk of atherosclerosis and hypertension in menopausal women.

Skin and Hair Health

Oestrogen is essential for maintaining skin elasticity, hydration, and thickness by boosting collagen production and preventing degradation. Declining oestrogen during menopause often leads to dry, sagging skin and thinning hair. Phytoestrogens, such as soy isoflavones and red clover, may counteract these effects by stimulating collagen synthesis, improving skin hydration, and reducing fine lines. These compounds may also nourish hair follicles, reducing hair thinning and promoting scalp health.

Mood and Brain Health

Menopause is associated with mood swings, depression, and mild cognitive decline due to reduced oestrogen levels. Phytoestrogens may exert neuroprotective effects by modulating brain receptors and boosting serotonin activity. While their impact is generally mild, studies suggest they can help stabilise mood and support memory retention. Regular intake of phytoestrogen-rich foods may contribute to better emotional well-being and cognitive health in menopausal women

Sources of Phytoestrogens

Phytoestrogens are found in many plant-based foods. Key sources include:

- **Isoflavones** (found in soy products like tofu, soy milk, and edamame).
- **Lignans** (present in flaxseeds, sesame seeds, whole grains, and berries).
- **Coumestans** (found in sprouts like alfalfa and clover).
- **Other foods**: Legumes (e.g., chickpeas), nuts, seeds, and some fruits and vegetables.

Evidence and Effectiveness

- While some studies have shown benefits of phytoestrogens for menopausal symptoms, the results are inconsistent. Factors such as diet, gut microbiota, and genetic differences may influence their effectiveness.
- Phytoestrogens are generally more effective in populations that consume

them regularly (e.g., Asian populations with soy-rich diets).

- Phytoestrogens may not work as strongly as Hormone Replacement Therapy (HRT), but they are a natural and accessible alternative for many women

Who Should Be Cautious with Phyto-oestrogenic Foods?

Phyto-oestrogens can mimic oestrogen in the body, they should be approached thoughtfully, especially for individuals with specific hormone-sensitive conditions like breast cancer or uterine fibroids.

People with Oestrogen-Sensitive Conditions:

Those with hormone-sensitive cancers (e.g., breast cancer) should consult with a healthcare professional before incorporating significant amounts of phyto-oestrogenic foods.

Those on Hormone Therapy:

If you are on hormone replacement therapy (HRT) or other medications that alter hormone levels, it is important to discuss phyto-oestrogen consumption with your doctor to avoid any interference with your treatment.

4 Low-Allergen, Low-Histamine Phytoestrogen Foods

For some women, menopause can exacerbate sensitivities to allergens and histamines, leading to additional discomfort.

Low-Allergen Foods

During menopause, the immune system can become more reactive due to hormonal fluctuations, which may heighten sensitivities or trigger food allergies. Common allergens like dairy, gluten, and certain nuts may become problematic. Low-allergen foods may help reduce the risk of inflammation and allergic reactions and reduce risks of gut disturbances and inflammatory responses, which can often worsen menopause symptoms such as bloating, digestive issues, or skin rashes.

Low-Histamine Foods

Histamine is a compound involved in immune responses and plays a role in the body's inflammatory reactions. Foods highest in histamine typically include fermented foods like aged cheeses, sauerkraut, as well as smoked or cured meats like salami and sausage. During menopause, histamine intolerance can become more prevalent due to changes in oestrogen metabolism. Oestrogen influences the enzymes that break down histamine, and a decline in oestrogen levels can cause a build-up of histamine, leading to symptoms like headaches, skin rashes, digestive upset, and even mood disturbances.

Low-histamine foods can help alleviate these symptoms by preventing the accumulation of excess histamine in the body. Foods that are fresh and minimally processed are typically low in histamine, while fermented foods, aged cheeses, and certain alcohols are high in histamine and may trigger flare-ups.

Table 1 below presents foods in descending order of phyto-oestrogenic activity based on the concentration and potency of their oestrogen-mimicking compounds. This ranking considers the known levels of phyto-oestrogens, their bioavailability, and their relative potency.

Table 1
Dietary Phytoestrogens and Relative Bioactivity ([A] Potential allergen)

Food/Herb	Phytoestrogenic Activity
Soybeans/Soy Products [A]	Highest phytoestrogenic activity (Isoflavones)
Flaxseeds	High phytoestrogenic activity (Lignans)
Red Clover Sprouts	High (Isoflavones, Formononetin, Biochanin A)
Hops	High (Xanthohumol, Isoflavones)
Fenugreek	Moderate (Saponins, Flavonoids)
Fennel	Moderate (Anethole, Oestrogenic)
Sesame Seeds [A]	Moderate (Lignans)
Pumpkin Seeds [A]	Moderate (Lignans, Omega-3s)
Sunflower Seeds [A]	Moderate (Lignans)
Broccoli and Broccoli Sprouts	Moderate (Indole-3-Carbinol, Oestrogen

Food/Herb	Phytoestrogenic Activity
	Metabolism)
Quinoa	Moderate (Lignans, Phytoestrogens)
Hibiscus	Moderate (Anthocyanins, flavonoids, phytoestrogens)
Lavender	Low to Moderate (Flavonoids, phytoestrogens)
Green Beans	Mild (Phytoestrogens)
Sweet Potatoes	Mild (Genistein, Phytoestrogens)
Plums (Prunes)	Mild (Lignans)
Sage	Mild phytoestrogen
Seaweed (Wakame, Nori|)	Mild (Fucoidan, Phytonutrients)
Apples	Low (Flavonoids, Mild Oestrogenic Activity)
Peaches	Low (Flavonoids, Mild Oestrogenic Activity)
Blueberries	Low (Flavonoids, Mild Oestrogenic Activity)

Food/Herb	Phytoestrogenic Activity
Red Grapes	Low (Resveratrol, Mild Phytoestrogenic Activity)
Cranberries	Low (Flavonoids, Mild Oestrogenic Activity)
Kiwi	Low (Flavonoids, Mild Oestrogenic Activity)
Cucumber	Low (Phytoestrogens)
Beets	Low (Phytoestrogens)
Avocado	Low (Phytoestrogens, Healthy Fats)
White Button Mushrooms	Low (Phytoestrogens)
Zucchini	Low (Phytoestrogens)
Oats	Low (Avenanthramides, Phytoestrogens)
Rice Bran	Low (Lignans, Phytoestrogens)
Asparagus	Low (Phytoestrogens)
Parsley	Low (Flavonoids, Phytoestrogens)
Endive	Low (Phytoestrogens)
Pears	Low (Phytoestrogens)

A more detailed of phytoestrogen rich foods is provided **in Chapter 9** in alphabetical order.

However, before jumping in your apron, here some important considerations.

5 Important Considerations for Phytoestrogens

Optimal Processing Techniques

- Use gentle cooking methods (steaming, light toasting).
- Grind seeds before consumption to maximise nutrient release.
- Consume fermented products (e.g., tempeh, miso) to enhance bioavailability.
- Store foods in airtight containers to prevent oxidation or degradation.

What to Avoid:
- Overcooking, prolonged high temperatures, or frying.
- Long-term storage of processed foods (e.g., pre-packaged juices or canned legumes).
- Excessive processing that removes fibre or bioactive compounds.

Synergy with Other Nutrients

Certain vitamins and minerals can work synergistically with phytoestrogens to enhance their effectiveness. For example:

- Vitamin D: Supports hormonal balance and may work together with phytoestrogens in regulating oestrogen receptors.
- Magnesium: Crucial for muscle function, relaxation, and mood regulation, especially during menopause. It may also support the efficacy of phytoestrogens in managing symptoms like mood swings.
- B Vitamins (especially B6 and B12): These vitamins are important for energy and mood regulation and can support the hormonal balancing effects of phytoestrogens.

Tip: Ensure you are consuming a diet with adequate vitamins and minerals to support overall hormone function and maximise the benefits of phytoestrogens.

The Role of the Gut Microbiome

The gut microbiome plays a critical role in the metabolism of phytoestrogens, especially lignans and isoflavones. The gut bacteria can help to convert these compounds into their more active forms. Therefore, maintaining a healthy gut is important for the bioavailability of phytoestrogens.

- Probiotics (like yogurt, kimchi, kefir) and prebiotics (like fibrous vegetables and whole grains) can help support a healthy microbiome.
- Antibiotics or a poor diet (high in processed foods) may disrupt the gut flora, reducing the conversion of phytoestrogens.

Tip: Incorporate fermented foods and fibre into your diet to enhance the conversion of phytoestrogens and overall gut health.

Timing of Phytoestrogen Intake

The timing of when you consume phytoestrogens can also be important. Many women report that taking phytoestrogen-rich foods at certain times of the day (e.g., morning or evening) can affect how they feel.

- Morning: Some women prefer taking phytoestrogen supplements in the morning as part of their breakfast routine for sustained energy and mood throughout the day.
- Evening: For those with sleep disturbances or nighttime hot flashes, taking phytoestrogens before bed may offer relief.

Tip: Experiment with the timing of your phytoestrogen intake and observe how your body responds.

Individual Variability

It is important to recognise that the response to phytoestrogens can vary from person to person. Some individuals may notice significant benefits, while others may not experience the same level of relief. The genetic factors involved in how your body processes and responds to phytoestrogens are unique, and factors like your gut microbiome, overall health, and diet can influence the effects.

Tip: Be patient and open to experimenting with different phytoestrogen-rich foods and supplements and track your progress over time. Consider keeping a food and symptom diary to monitor how certain foods affect your menopausal symptoms.

Combining Phytoestrogens with Conventional Treatments

If you're undergoing hormone replacement therapy (HRT) or using bioidentical hormones, it is possible to combine these with phytoestrogen-rich foods to help manage symptoms. However, consulting with your healthcare provider is crucial, as they can help you incorporate both approaches safely.

Phytoestrogens in Food vs. Supplements

Many people wonder if they should opt for food sources of phytoestrogens (like soy, flaxseeds, and chickpeas) or supplements (e.g., soy isoflavones or red clover extracts). Food sources tend to provide a broader range of nutrients and may be a safer long-term option, while supplements can provide a concentrated dose but should be used with caution.

Tip: Prioritise getting your phytoestrogens from whole foods, and consider supplements, if necessary, but always under the guidance of a healthcare provider.

Long-Term Use and Safety

Although phytoestrogens are generally considered safe for most people, it is important to be mindful of long-term use. While they are often considered less potent than synthetic oestrogens, there is still some ongoing research into their long-term effects and their impact on conditions like breast cancer or endometriosis.

6 Dietary Components

Certain dietary components and lifestyle factors can interfere with the absorption or bioavailability of phytoestrogens, potentially reducing their effectiveness or making them less beneficial. Here's a summary of what to avoid maximizing the bioavailability and effectiveness of phytoestrogen-rich foods and supplements.

High-Fat Diets (Especially Saturated Fats)

High levels of saturated fats (found in fatty meats, full-fat dairy, processed oils, and some baked goods) can reduce the absorption of phytoestrogens, especially lignans (from flaxseeds, sesame seeds, etc.). These fats may also interfere with the conversion of certain phytoestrogens into their bioactive forms in the body.

Tips: Try to avoid excessive saturated fats, and focus on healthy fats (e.g., those from avocado, nuts, seeds, and olive oil), which are less likely to inhibit phytoestrogen absorption.

Caffeine

Caffeine, found in coffee, tea, chocolate, and some drinks, can interfere with the metabolism of phytoestrogens like isoflavones (from soy) and lignans. Caffeine may also affect the gut microbiome, which plays a role in the conversion of certain phytoestrogens (like those in flaxseeds and soy) into more bioactive forms. Caffein can also impact sleep.

Tips: The literature highlights some of the benefits of coffee, they key here is "moderation": Limit caffeine intake, especially in the hours surrounding the consumption of phytoestrogen-rich foods. If you consume caffeine, do not exceed 2 cups a day, try to avoid it with meals and 6 hours before bedtime.

Alcohol

Alcohol can impair the liver's ability to process phytoestrogens effectively, reducing their bioavailability. Additionally, alcohol consumption can disrupt the gut microbiota, which plays a role in phytoestrogen metabolism.

Tips Limit alcohol intake, especially for those who are using phytoestrogen-rich foods or supplements for menopause symptom relief. If consumed, do so in moderation.

High Amounts of Calcium and Iron (from Supplements or Certain Foods)

High amounts of calcium (found in dairy and fortified foods) and iron (especially from supplements) can bind to phytoestrogens like isoflavones (from soy) and reduce their absorption. This can especially be a concern when consuming calcium supplements or iron-rich foods at the same time as phytoestrogenic meals.

Tips: Try to separate the intake of calcium or iron supplements from phytoestrogen-rich foods by a few hours and avoid consuming foods with high calcium or iron content at the same time.

Soy Protein Isolate (and Other Highly Processed Soy Products)

While soy products are a rich source of phytoestrogens, processed soy protein isolates (found in many processed and vegetarian foods) may lower the bioavailability of isoflavones due to their processing methods. The refining process can reduce the concentration of active phytoestrogen compounds, and some added chemicals in processed soy can interfere with the body's absorption of nutrients.

Tips: Choose whole soy foods like tofu, tempeh, edamame, and organic soy milk over heavily processed soy isolates.

High Sugar Diets

Diets high in refined sugars (e.g., white bread, pastries, drinks) can disrupt gut health, leading to poor absorption of phytoestrogens and a decrease in their beneficial effects. Elevated blood sugar can also contribute to inflammation, which may counteract the beneficial effects of phytoestrogens

Tips: Minimise intake of refined sugars and focus on whole foods with a low glycaemic index (e.g., vegetables, whole grains, fruits in moderation).

Protein, Not Any Protein

While lean red meat can provide protein and iron, high consumption—particularly of processed meat—has well-documented health drawbacks, especially in midlife women.

Harmful Compounds: Haem and Nitrosamines
Red meat contains haem, which, in high amounts, can cause oxidative stress and inflammation. Processed meats often contain nitrites and nitrates, which can form nitrosamines, compounds linked to increased risk of colorectal, breast, and other cancers.

Salt and Preservatives
Processed meats are also high in salt (sodium), added as a preservative and flavour enhancer. Excess sodium intake is a major contributor to high blood pressure, which becomes more common after menopause. Salt also contributes to fluid retention, bloating, and may worsen bone loss by increasing calcium

excretion. Additionally, chemical preservatives like sodium nitrite and phosphates may negatively affect kidney and vascular health when consumed frequently.

Heart and Vascular Health
High intake of saturated fats and preservatives in red and processed meat contributes to plaque buildup in arteries, raising the risk of heart attacks and strokes—already elevated in postmenopausal women.

Bone and Kidney Strain
Diets high in animal protein and salt can raise the body's acid load, increasing calcium loss from bones. Over time, this may weaken bone structure and strain the kidneys, particularly in women who are already at risk of bone density loss.

Weight and Metabolic Control
Processed meats are often calorie-dense, high in unhealthy fats, and low in fibre. This combination is unfavourable for weight management and is associated with increased insulin resistance and inflammation, both linked to metabolic dysfunction.

Tips: A high **plant-protein, low red meat** diet is a powerful nutritional approach for women navigating perimenopause and menopause. It supports hormonal balance, protects the heart and bones, aids in healthy weight maintenance, and helps prevent chronic diseases. At the same time, reducing red and processed meat minimizes exposure to harmful compounds like nitrosamines, haem, preservatives, and excess salt, all of which can undermine health during this vulnerable life stage.

Encouraging the inclusion of more legumes, nuts, tofu, tempeh, seeds, and whole grains, while cutting back on bacon, sausages, deli meats, and other processed items, can make a meaningful difference in long-term well-being.

Medications and Herbal Supplements

Some medications, like those used for thyroid issues or antibiotics, may affect gut bacteria and reduce the body's ability to convert and absorb phytoestrogens. Additionally, herbal supplements like St. John's Wort and ginseng may interfere with hormonal pathways or the absorption of phytoestrogens.

Tips: Always consult a healthcare provider when adding phytoestrogen-rich foods or supplements, especially if you're on medications or other supplements that might interfere with their absorption or metabolism.

A list of herbals/nutraceuticals is provided in Chapter 13.

7 Physical Activity and Sleep

Physical activity, sports and sleep can have a significant impact on wellbeing, physically and emotionally.

Physical activity guidelines:[1,2]

- At least 150 minutes of moderate intensity (cycling, brisk walking, swimming) per week
- OR at least 75 minutes of vigorous intensity (running, sports) per week
- Building muscle strength (carrying shopping, gym, yoga) at least 2 days/week
- Working on balance (dancing, Tai chi)
- Seven hours sleep or more per night

[1] Officers, U. C. M. (2019). UK chief medical officers' physical activity guidelines. United Kingdom Department of Health and Social Care, Llwodraeth Cymru Welsh Government, Department of Health Northern Ireland and the Scottish Government.

[2] Bull FC, Al-Ansari SS, Biddle S, et al., (2020). World Health Organization 2020 guidelines on physical activity and sedentary behaviour British Journal of Sports Medicine, 54(24),1451-1462

Physical Activity & Exercise in menopause

Regular physical activity, particularly weight-bearing and aerobic exercises, can help regulate hormonal balance, and reduce stress. Exercise has been shown to increase the sensitivity of oestrogen receptors, meaning your body may respond better to the oestrogenic effects of phytoestrogens when combined with regular exercise.

- Weight training can help boost bone health (which can decline during menopause) and improve overall hormone balance.
- Yoga and meditation can help manage stress, which is crucial for overall hormonal health.

Tip: Incorporate regular exercise into your routine to support the effectiveness of phytoestrogens and improve overall health during menopause. It may be a good time to join a gym, a regular class, or recruit a personal trainer for one-to-one tailored support.

Physical Activities Suitable for Menopause

Aqua Aerobics: Low-impact water-based exercises that improve cardiovascular health and are easy on joints.

Barre: Combines elements of ballet, yoga, and Pilates; great for muscle toning and balance.

Cycling: Low-impact cardio that supports joint health and cardiovascular fitness.

Dancing: A fun activity that boosts mood while improving balance and bone density.

Elliptical Training: Provides low-impact cardio, beneficial for heart health and weight management.

Gardening: A gentle physical activity that reduces stress and strengthens muscles.

Hiking: Combines weight-bearing exercise for bone health with nature's calming effects.

Pilates: Strengthens core muscles, improves

posture, and enhances flexibility.

Resistance Band Workouts: Builds muscle strength and supports joint health in a gentle way.

Strength Training or Gym Workouts: Builds muscle mass and improves bone density.

Swimming: A low-impact exercise that is gentle on joints and improves cardiovascular health.

Tai Chi: A gentle, flowing martial art that reduces stress, improves balance, and supports joint health.

Walking: An accessible, weight-bearing exercise that supports bone and cardiovascular health.

Yoga: Reduces stress, improves flexibility, and aids in managing hot flashes and sleep issues.

Zumba: Combines fun dance routines with cardio and balance training, great for mood and fitness.

Sleep

Sleep is a crucial process in bodily repair

and the processing of information. The consequences of poor sleep include exacerbation of mental health disorders, impaired concentration and memory, increased poor/ risky decision making and an increased risk of injuries and obesity.[1, 2]

[1]McMain, S., Newman, M. G., Segal, Z. V., & DeRubeis, R. J. (2015). Cognitive behavioral therapy: Current status and future research directions. *Psychotherapy Research*, *25*(3), 321–329. https://doi.org/10.1080/10503307.2014.1002440

[2]Riemann, D., Baglioni, C., Bassetti, C.. . . Spiegelhalder, K. (2017). European guideline for the diagnosis and treatment of insomnia. *Journal of Sleep Research*, *26*(6), 675–700. https://doi.org/10.1111/jsr.12594

Creative, Relaxation, Stress Busting Activities that may help with Sleep

- Aromatherapy
- Baking & cooking
- Beauty, facial, brows, lashes
- Bird watching
- Board games
- Card games
- Concert
- Counselling
- Crochet

- Drawing
- Exposition & gallery
- Flower arranging
- Fishing
- Hairdresser
- Jewellery making
- Journaling or creative writing
- Knitting
- Learning a language
- Macrame
- Manicure & pedicure
- Massage
- Meditation
- Miniatures
- Museum
- Music playing & listening
- Painting
- Pet sitting
- Pottery
- Reflexology
- Sculpting
- Spa day
- Upholstery
- Volunteering

8 Environmental Factors That Disrupt Hormones

Environmental factors, particularly endocrine-disrupting chemicals (EDCs), can interfere with hormone function and disrupt the delicate hormonal balance, especially during menopause. These disruptors can mimic, block, or interfere with the natural action of hormones like oestrogen, leading to various health issues. Below are some common environmental factors that may disrupt hormones and advice for menopausal women:

Common Hormone Disruptors

Phthalates (found in plastics, perfumes, cosmetics)

- o Effect: Can mimic oestrogen, disrupt the endocrine system, and affect reproductive health.
- o Advice: Minimise use of plastic containers, especially for food and drink.

- o Tip: Opt for phthalate-free beauty and cleaning products.

Bisphenol A (BPA) (found in some plastics and food cans)

- o Effect: Known as an oestrogen-mimicking chemical. It can increase the risk of hormonal imbalances.

- o Tip: Choose BPA-free products, avoid canned food where possible, and opt for glass or stainless-steel containers.

Parabens (found in personal care products like lotions, shampoos, deodorants)

- o Effect: Parabens can mimic oestrogen and may contribute to hormone disruption.

- o Tip: Use paraben-free cosmetics and personal care products. Look for natural alternatives.

Pesticides and Herbicides (found in non-organic produce)

- o Effect: Certain pesticides, like glyphosate, can act as endocrine disruptors.

- o Tip Opt for organic produce where possible to reduce exposure to these chemicals.

Heavy Metals (lead, mercury, cadmium)
- o Effect: Can affect hormone synthesis and disrupt metabolic functions.

- o Tip Avoid exposure to sources of heavy metals (e.g., old paint, contaminated water, certain seafood) and prioritise natural detoxification methods.

Flame Retardants (found in furniture, electronics, mattresses)
- o Effect: Flame retardants can mimic thyroid and oestrogen hormones, affecting hormone balance.

- o Tip: Look for flame-retardant-free

furniture and ensure your living spaces are well-ventilated to avoid buildup of these chemicals.
- o to minimise exposure.

Artificial Sweeteners (like aspartame, sucralose)
- o Effect: Some studies suggest artificial sweeteners might affect insulin and disrupt hormonal balance.

- o Tip: Limit the intake of artificial sweeteners and opt for natural sweeteners like stevia or honey when necessary.

Endocrine Disrupting Chemicals in Air and Water Pollution
- o Effect: Pollutants can affect hormone production, particularly thyroid function.

- o Tip: Reduce exposure by staying indoors on high pollution days, using air purifiers, and avoiding smoking or second-hand smoke.

General Advice for Menopausal Women to Minimise Hormonal Disruptors:

- Grow some of your own foods organically (herbs, leafy greens cn be produced in windows in small spaces).
- Buy and eat organic foods reduce pesticide and herbicide exposure.
- Avoid plastic containers for food storage and drinking (use glass, stainless steel, or bamboo).
- Switch to natural beauty products free from phthalates, parabens, and synthetic fragrances.
- Chose toxin-free cleaning products, using a water filter, and opting for non-toxic furniture and mattresses. Instead use natural soaps and hot water, and blends of white vinegars and sodium bicarbonates with essential oils.
- Incorporate foods like cruciferous vegetables (broccoli, cauliflower, kale) to support the liver in processing toxins.
- Reduce exposure to endocrine-disrupting chemicals, avoid non-organic meat and dairy, as they may contain residues from hormones or antibiotics.

9 Phytoestrogenic Foods

Foods containing phytoestrogens are detailed in alphabetical order below.

Alfalfa Sprouts
- Active Compound: Coumestrol
- Bioactive Dose: 20-50 g of fresh sprouts daily.
- Time to See Effects: Noticeable effects within a month of daily intake.
- Preparation/Processing:
  - Best: Consume raw or lightly steamed. Sprouting maximises coumestrol content.
  - Avoid: Overcooking or prolonged exposure to sunlight after harvesting.

Anise and Fennel Seeds
- Active Compound: Anethole
- Bioactive Dose: ~1-2 teaspoons (2-4 g) daily.
- Time to See Effects: Varies, but consistent use over 2-4 weeks is recommended.

- Preparation/Processing:
    - Best: Use in teas or lightly toast before grinding.

Avoid: Over-roasting or exposing to humid conditions, which can degrade potency.

Apples
- Active Compound: Phloridzin (a flavonoid with weak oestrogenic activity)
- Bioactive Dose: 1-2 medium apples (~200 g) daily.
- Time to See Effects: Gradual benefits after 6-8 weeks of daily consumption.
- Preparation/Processing:
    - Best: Eat raw with the peel for maximum flavonoid content.
    - Avoid: Peeling or cooking at high temperatures, which degrade phloridzin.

Asparagus
- Active Compound: Saponins (mild oestrogenic effect).
- Bioactive Dose: ~1 cup cooked (~150 g) daily.
- Time to See Effects: Benefits over 6-8 weeks of consistent intake.

- Preparation/Processing:
  - Best: Steam or roast lightly.
  - Avoid: Boiling for extended periods, which can deplete nutrients.

Avocado
- Active Compound: Phytosterols (support oestrogen metabolism).
- Bioactive Dose: ~½ medium avocado (~75 g) daily.
- Time to See Effects: Gradual effects over 6-8 weeks.
- Preparation/Processing:
  - Best: Eat raw or add to smoothies.
  - Avoid: Cooking at high temperatures, which affects oils.

Beets
- Active Compound: Betalains (indirect oestrogenic effects)
- Bioactive Dose: 1 medium beet (~100-150 g) daily.
- Time to See Effects: Gradual benefits over 4-6 weeks.
- Preparation/Processing:

- Best: Roast or steam to retain nutrients.

Avoid: Prolonged boiling, which leaches betalains.

Blueberries
- Active Compound: Flavonoids (e.g., Quercetin)
- Bioactive Dose: ½ cup (~75 g) daily.
- Time to See Effects: Gradual benefits over 6-8 weeks.
- Preparation/Processing:
    - Best: Consume fresh or in smoothies.
    - Avoid: Baking at high temperatures, which can reduce flavonoid content.

Broccoli and Broccoli Sprouts
- Active Compound: Isoflavones and sulforaphane (indirect oestrogen modulator)
- Bioactive Dose: ~1 cup cooked broccoli or ½ cup sprouts daily.
- Time to See Effects: 4-6 weeks of regular intake.
- Preparation/Processing:

- Best: Lightly steam to maximise sulforaphane and isoflavone content.
- Avoid
  - Microwaving for too long, which destroys sulforaphane.
  - High consumption of broccoli with low thyroid function due to the presence of goitrogens.

Carrots
- Active Compound: Beta-carotene (weak oestrogenic activity)
- Bioactive Dose: ~1 medium carrot (50-70 g) daily.
- Time to See Effects: Gradual benefits over 8-12 weeks.
- Preparation/Processing:
  - Best: Steam or eat raw to preserve beta-carotene.
  - Avoid: Overboiling, which reduces nutrient content.

Chickpeas (and other legumes)
- Active Compound: Isoflavones

- Bioactive Dose: ~50 mg of isoflavones from ~1 cup (160 g) cooked chickpeas per day.
- Time to See Effects: 6-8 weeks of regular consumption.
- Preparation/Processing:
- Best: Soak and cook thoroughly to reduce antinutrients.
- Avoid: Canned chickpeas stored for long periods may lose some phyto-oestrogen activity.

Cloves

- Active Compound: Eugenol (a potent antioxidant) and phytoestrogenic compounds.
- Bioactive Dose:
- ½ to 1 teaspoon of ground cloves daily.
- Alternatively, 1-2 whole cloves steeped in tea.
- Time to See Effects: 4-6 weeks of regular consumption for noticeable benefits in managing oxidative stress and mild hormonal support.
- Preparation/Processing:

- Best: Use ground cloves in baking, curries, or smoothies.
- Add whole cloves to teas, soups, or stews and simmer to extract active compounds.
- Avoid: Overheating cloves for extended periods, which can degrade eugenol.

Courgette/Zucchini
- Active Compound: Lutein and flavonoids.
- Bioactive Dose: 1 cup cooked zucchini (~150 g) daily.
- Time to See Effects: Gradual benefits in 6-8 weeks.
- Preparation/Processing:
  - Best: Steam or sauté lightly.
  - Avoid: Overcooking, which depletes nutrients.

Cranberries
- Active Compound: Flavonoids (e.g., Quercetin) and proanthocyanidins.
- Bioactive Dose: ~½ cup fresh or 1/4 cup dried cranberries daily.
- Time to See Effects: Gradual benefits over 6-8 weeks.

- Preparation/Processing:
  - Best: Consume fresh or dried with no added sugar.
  - Avoid: High-sugar cranberry juice cocktails.

Cucumber
- Active Compound: Cucurbitacins (mild phyto-oestrogenic and anti-inflammatory activity).
- Bioactive Dose: ~1 medium cucumber (~150 g) daily.
- Time to See Effects: Subtle effects over 6-8 weeks.
- Preparation/Processing:
  - Best: Eat raw with the peel to maximise phytonutrient content.
  - Avoid: Peeling or cooking, which reduces bioactivity.

Endive
- Active Compound: Flavonoids and saponins.
- Bioactive Dose: ~1 cup raw or ½ cup cooked (~50-100 g) daily.
- Time to See Effects: 4-6 weeks.
- Preparation/Processing:

- Best: Use fresh in salads or lightly sauté.
- Avoid: Overcooking, which reduces phytonutrient content.

Fennel seeds
- Active Compound: Anethole (phytoestrogenic, antioxidant, and anti-inflammatory properties).
- Bioactive Dose: 1–2 teaspoons of fennel seeds daily. For medicinal purposes, fennel tea (1 teaspoon of seeds in hot water) can be consumed 1–2 times daily.
- Time to See Effects:
- Hormonal Balance: 4–6 weeks.
- Digestive Relief: Benefits noticeable within a few days.
- Preparation/Processing:
  - Best: Use fennel seeds in teas, ground into powder for smoothies, or as a spice in cooking.
  - Brew fennel tea by steeping 1 teaspoon of seeds in hot water for 5–10 minutes.
  - Avoid:
  - Overheating seeds for extended periods, as it degrades anethole.

- Excessive intake, which may cause hormonal imbalances or digestive discomfort.

Fenugreek
- Active Compound: Diosgenin (a phyto-oestrogen precursor), trigonelline, and saponins.
- Bioactive Dose:
    - Fenugreek seeds: ~2-5 grams (½-1 teaspoon) per day.
    - Fenugreek tea: Brewed from ~1-2 teaspoons (2-4 g) of seeds.
    - Fenugreek supplements: Follow manufacturer guidelines (commonly 500-1000 mg/day).
- Time to See Effects: Hormonal balancing effects typically noticed in 4-6 weeks.
- Preparation/Processing:
    - Best:
        - Soak seeds overnight and consume raw or lightly cooked to retain active compounds.

- Use in teas: Simmer seeds for 10-15 minutes to extract bioactive compounds.
- As a spice: Lightly toast before grinding for flavour but avoid over-toasting.
- Avoid:
  - Excessive heating or boiling for long periods, which degrades diosgenin and saponins.
  - Long-term storage in humid conditions, which reduces potency

Fenugreek's diosgenin is particularly significant because it acts as a precursor to oestrogen-like compounds and has been studied for its potential to alleviate menopausal symptoms, enhance lactation, and support hormonal balance. Its saponins also contribute to oestrogenic effects and provide additional benefits like reducing inflammation and improving metabolic health.

Green Beans
- Active Compound: Isoflavones and lignans
- Bioactive Dose: 1 cup (~100-150 g) daily.
- Time to See Effects: Effects can appear after 4-6 weeks.
- Preparation/Processing:
    - Best: Steam or sauté lightly.
    - Avoid: Overboiling, which depletes bioactive compounds.

Hibiscus
- Active Compound: Anthocyanins, Flavonoids (e.g., quercetin, kaempferol), Phytoestrogens
- Bioactive Dose: 1-2 cups of tea (around 5-10 grams of dried hibiscus flowers) per day.
- Time to See Effects: 1-2 weeks of regular use.
- Preparation/Processing:
    - Best: Steep dried flowers in hot water to make tea. Can also be added to smoothies or incorporated into desserts for flavour and health benefits.

- Avoid: Boiling for prolonged periods, as it may degrade some of the active compounds and reduce potency.

Hops (e.g., Hops Tea or Extracts)
- Active Compound: 8-Prenylnaringenin (a potent phyto-oestrogen)
- Bioactive Dose: ~0.5-1 mg of 8-prenylnaringenin per day (approximately 1-2 cups of hops tea or supplements as per manufacturer instructions).
- Time to See Effects: Can be effective within 2-4 weeks.
- Preparation/Processing:
    - Best: Brew as tea (steep 1-2 g dried hops in boiling water for 5-10 minutes).
    - Avoid: Excessive heating or prolonged storage of dried hops.

Kiwi

- Active Compound: Flavonoids and vitamin C (supporting oestrogen metabolism).
- Bioactive Dose: 1-2 kiwis (~100-200 g) daily.

- Time to See Effects: Benefits in 4-6 weeks.
- Preparation/Processing:
    - Best: Eat fresh with the peel (if washed and organic).
    - Avoid: Juicing, which removes fibre and some nutrients.

Lavender
- Active Compound: Flavonoids (e.g., apigenin, luteolin), Phytoestrogens (in small amounts)
- Bioactive Dose: 1-2 teaspoons of dried lavender flowers (around 1-2 grams) per day, typically in tea.
- Time to See Effects: 1-2 weeks of regular use, depending on individual sensitivity.
- Preparation/Processing:
    - Best: Steep dried flowers in hot water for tea, or use in aromatherapy (e.g., lavender essential oil) to promote relaxation and hormonal balance.
    - Avoid: High-heat methods of extraction (e.g., prolonged boiling), as this can diminish the

beneficial effects of lavender's essential oils and flavonoids.

Nuts (Almonds, Walnuts)
- Active Compound: Lignans and polyphenols
- Bioactive Dose: ~20-30 g (1 small handful) daily.
- Time to See Effects: Gradual benefits over 6-8 weeks.
- Preparation/Processing:
    - Best: Consume raw or lightly toasted.
    - Avoid: Roasting at high temperatures for extended periods.
    - <u>Avoid</u> with nut allergies

Plums (Dried as Prunes)
- Active Compound: Flavonoids (e.g., Chlorogenic Acid)
- Bioactive Dose: ~3-5 prunes (30-50 g) daily.
- Time to See Effects: Noticeable in 6-8 weeks.
- Preparation/Processing:

- Best: Consume dried or soaked in water overnight.
- Avoid: Excessive processing with sugar or additives.

Oats

- Active Compound: Avenanthramides (antioxidant polyphenols with oestrogenic effects)
- Bioactive Dose: ~½-1 cup (40-80 g) of oats daily.
- Time to See Effects: Consistent benefits in 6-8 weeks.
- Preparation/Processing:
  - Best: Cook as oatmeal or soak overnight.
  - Avoid: High-sugar or processed instant oats.

Parsley

- Active Compound: Apigenin (a flavonoid with oestrogenic properties)
- Bioactive Dose: ~5-10 g of fresh parsley daily.
- Time to See Effects: Consistent intake over 6-8 weeks.
- Preparation/Processing:

- Best: Add fresh to salads, soups, or smoothies.
- Avoid: Overcooking, which reduces flavonoid content.

Peaches
- Active Compound: Lignans and flavonoids (e.g., Naringenin)
- Bioactive Dose: 1 medium peach (~150 g) daily.
- Time to See Effects: Effects may be observed after 6-8 weeks.
- Preparation/Processing:
  - Best: Consume fresh or lightly poached.
  - Avoid: Canned peaches in syrup or overcooking, which reduce flavonoid content.

Pear
- Active Compound: Flavonoids (e.g., Phloretin).
- Bioactive Dose: 1 medium pear (~150 g) daily.
- Time to See Effects: Subtle effects in 6-8 weeks.
- Preparation/Processing:
  - Best: Eat raw with the peel.

- Avoid: Peeling or cooking extensively.

Pomegranates
- Active Compound: Ellagitannins (converted to urolithins in the gut)
- Bioactive Dose: ½ to 1 cup (125-250 ml) of fresh juice or arils daily.
- Time to See Effects: After 4-8 weeks of regular intake.
- Preparation/Processing:
    - Best: Consume fresh juice or arils. Light blending can release compounds.
    - Avoid: Store-bought juices with added sugar and prolonged storage, which degrade nutrients.

Pumpkin Seeds
- Active Compound: Lignans and zinc (indirectly supports oestrogen receptor function)
- Bioactive Dose: ~1-2 tablespoons (15-30 g) daily.
- Time to See Effects: 4-6 weeks of regular consumption.
- Preparation/Processing:

- Best: Lightly roast or consume raw.
- Avoid: Prolonged heating or exposure to light, which degrade nutrients.

Quinoa
- Active Compound: Flavonoids (Quercetin, Kaempferol)
- Bioactive Dose: 1 cup cooked quinoa (~185 g) daily.
- Time to See Effects: Gradual benefits after 6-8 weeks.
- Preparation/Processing:
    - Best: Cook with minimal water to preserve flavonoids.
    - Avoid: Overcooking or reheating repeatedly.

Red Grapes
- Active Compound: Resveratrol and flavonoids.
- Bioactive Dose: ~1 cup fresh grapes (~150 g) or ½ cup grape juice daily.
- Time to See Effects: 4-6 weeks.
- Preparation/Processing:
    - Best: Consume fresh or as juice.

- Avoid: Fermented or alcoholic forms (e.g., wine), which can be high in histamines.

Red Clover Sprouts
- Active Compound: Isoflavones (Biochanin A, Formononetin)
- Bioactive Dose: 40-80 mg/day (from ~50-100 g sprouts daily).
- Time to See Effects: Noticeable effects in 4-6 weeks.
- Preparation/Processing:
    - Best: Consume fresh or lightly steamed. Sprouting enhances isoflavone content.

Avoid: Excessive heating or prolonged storage after sprouting, which reduces isoflavone content.

Rice Bran
- Active Compound: Gamma-oryzanol (plant sterol with oestrogenic properties).
- Bioactive Dose: ~1 tablespoon (~10 g) daily.
- Time to See Effects: 4-6 weeks of regular intake.
- Preparation/Processing:

- Best: Sprinkle onto oatmeal, yogurt, or smoothies.
- Avoid: High-heat processing, which destroys oryzanol content.

Sage (Salvia officinalis)
- Active Compound: Rosmarinic acid, luteolin, apigenin, camphor, and thujone.
- Bioactive Dose:
  - Tea: 1-2 cups of sage tea (2-3 grams of dried sage leaves) daily.
  - Topical Use: Sage-infused oil or diluted essential oil (3-5 drops in a carrier oil) applied to the scalp to support hair health and reduce hot flashes.
- Time to See Effects: 1-2 weeks for hot flash reduction; 6-8 weeks for scalp benefits.
- Preparation/Processing:
  - Best:
    - Steep dried sage leaves in hot water for tea.
    - Use sage-infused oil for scalp massages or skin applications.
    - Incorporate fresh sage into meals for added health benefits.

- o Avoid:
  - ▪ Overuse of sage essential oil, as the high thujone content can be toxic in large quantities.
  - ▪ Prolonged boiling of sage leaves, which may degrade beneficial compounds.

Seaweed (e.g., Wakame, Nori)
- Active Compound: Lignans and iodine (essential for hormonal balance).
- Bioactive Dose: ~5-10 g dried seaweed daily (amounts vary by iodine content).
- Time to See Effects: Hormonal effects in 6-8 weeks.
- Preparation/Processing:
  - Best: Add to soups, salads, or eat as sheets (nori).
  - Avoid: Over-soaking or boiling for too long, which reduces bioactive compounds.

Sesame Seeds
- Active Compound: Lignans (Sesamin, Sesamolin)
- Bioactive Dose: 1-2 tablespoons (15-30 g) daily.

- Time to See Effects: 4-6 weeks of regular use.
- Preparation/Processing:
  - Best: Toast seeds lightly or use as tahini paste to enhance digestibility and bioavailability.
  - Avoid: High-temperature roasting for extended periods.

Soy Products
- Active Compound: Isoflavones (Genistein, Daidsein)
- Bioactive Dose: 50-100 mg/day is considered effective.
- Time to See Effects: Effects may appear after 4-6 weeks of consistent consumption.
- Preparation/Processing:
  - Best: Fermented soy products like tempeh or miso enhance isoflavone bioavailability. Soy milk and tofu also retain bioactivity.
  - Avoid: Overheating (e.g., frying) or excessive processing can degrade isoflavones.

- Low-Histamine Considerations: Fresh tofu and non-aged soy milk are preferable to avoid histamine formation.

Sunflower Seeds
- Active Compound: Lignans and vitamin E (supportive of oestrogen pathways).
- Bioactive Dose: ~1-2 tablespoons (15-30 g) daily.
- Time to See Effects: Gradual improvement in 6-8 weeks.
- Preparation/Processing:
  - Best: Eat raw or lightly toasted.
  - Avoid: High-temperature roasting, which degrades vitamin E. Consume in moderation only.

Sweet Potatoes
- Active Compound: Diosgenin (a ic precursor)
- Bioactive Dose: ~150 g (1 medium sweet potato) daily.
- Time to See Effects: 6-8 weeks of daily intake.
- Preparation/Processing:
  - Best: Bake or steam.

Avoid: Frying or charring, which degrade bioactive compounds.

White Button Mushrooms
- Active Compound: Polysaccharides (indirect oestrogen modulators).
- Bioactive Dose: ~1 cup cooked (~100 g) daily.
- Time to See Effects: Subtle effects over 6-8 weeks.
- Preparation/Processing:
    - Best: Lightly sauté or steam.
    - Avoid: Overcooking or frying.

10 One Day Food Diary Example

Here is a sample 24-hour food diary designed for a vegan menopausal woman, balancing macronutrients according to the recommended proportions (45% carbohydrates, 25% protein, and 30% fats).

This plan also focuses on foods rich in phytoestrogens, antioxidants, and anti-inflammatory compounds, which are beneficial during menopause.

Breakfast:
- Smoothie Bowl
    - 1/2 cup unsweetened almond milk (calcium and vitamin D)
    - 1 tablespoon ground flaxseeds (phytoestrogens, omega-3s)
    - 1 tablespoon chia seeds (fiber, omega-3s, lignans)
    - 1/2 frosen banana (fiber, potassium)
    - 1/2 cup blueberries (antioxidants)
    - 2 tablespoons almond butter (healthy fats, protein)

- ○ Toppings: Sliced almonds, chia seeds, and a sprinkle of hemp seeds

Hydration:

- 1 glass of water with lemon (vitamin C for immune support)

Energy and Nutrients:

- Calories: ~350 kcal
- Carbohydrates: ~40g (Fiber: 8g, Sugars: 15g)
- Protein: ~8g
- Fat: ~20g (Healthy fats from almond butter, flaxseeds, and chia seeds)

Mid-Morning Snack:

- Green Tea (rich in antioxidants)
- Handful of Walnuts (good source of omega-3 fatty acids and phytoestrogens)

Energy and Nutrients:

- Calories: ~200 kcal
- Carbohydrates: ~4g
- Protein: ~5g
- Fat: ~18g (High in omega-3 fatty acids)

Lunch:
- Lentil and Quinoa Salad
  - 1 cup cooked quinoa (complete protein and fiber)
  - 1/2 cup cooked lentils (rich in plant-based protein and fiber)
  - 1/2 cup chopped kale (calcium, antioxidants, phytoestrogens)
  - 1 tablespoon tahini (healthy fats, calcium, lignans)
  - 1/4 cup chopped cucumbers and tomatoes (hydration and vitamins)
  - Lemon-tahini dressing (1 tbsp tahini, lemon juice, olive oil, salt, pepper)

Hydration:
- 1 glass of water with a splash of apple cider vinegar (gut health)

Energy and Nutrients:
- Calories: ~500 kcal
- Carbohydrates: ~65g (Fiber: 15g, Sugars: 5g)
- Protein: ~22g
- Fat: ~20g (Healthy fats from tahini and olive oil)

Afternoon Snack:
- Soy Yogurt with Mixed Berries
    - 1/2 cup unsweetened soy yogurt (rich in isoflavones)
    - 1/2 cup mixed berries (antioxidants, vitamins)
    - 1 tablespoon hemp seeds (omega-3s, protein)

Hydration:
- 1 cup of water or herbal tea (peppermint or ginger)

Energy and Nutrients:
- Calories: ~150 kcal
- Carbohydrates: ~18g (Fiber: 5g, Sugars: 12g)
- Protein: ~7g
- Fat: ~8g

Dinner:
- Chickpea & Spinach Stew
    - 1 cup cooked chickpeas (high in protein and fiber)
    - 1/2 cup cooked spinach (iron, calcium, phytoestrogens)
    - 1/4 cup diced tomatoes (antioxidants, lycopene)

- o 1/2 tablespoon olive oil (healthy fats, anti-inflammatory)
- o Spices: Turmeric, cumin, garlic, black pepper
- o Serve with 1/2 cup cooked brown rice (fiber, magnesium)

Hydration:
- 1 glass of water or herbal tea (chamomile for relaxation)

Energy and Nutrients:
- Calories: ~500 kcal
- Carbohydrates: ~65g (Fiber: 16g, Sugars: 8g)
- Protein: ~20g
- Fat: ~15g (Healthy fats from olive oil)

Evening Snack:
- Dark Chocolate & Almonds
  - o 2-3 squares of dark chocolate (70% or more; rich in antioxidants)
  - o 1 small handful of almonds (healthy fats, protein, vitamin E)

Hydration:
- 1 glass of water or warm herbal tea (such as ginger or lemon balm)

Energy and Nutrients:
- Calories: ~200 kcal
- Carbohydrates: ~15g (Fiber: 4g, Sugars: 10g)
- Protein: ~5g
- Fat: ~16g

Total Estimated Daily Intake:
- Calories: ~**1,900 kcal**
- Carbohydrates: ~207g (Fiber: 48g, Sugars: 50g)
- Protein: ~67g
- Fat: ~80g

Now for some of my favourite recipes…

11 Cooking Recipes

Meno Floral Tea Blend

Ingredients:
- 1 tablespoon dried Hibiscus flowers (for oestrogenic support, antioxidants, and hot flash relief)
- 1 tablespoon dried Chamomile flower (for calming and sleep support)
- 1 tablespoon dried Lavender flowers (for relaxation and hormonal balance)
- 1 tablespoon dried Red Clover flower (for phytoestrogens to help with hot flashes and bone health)
- 1 teaspoon dried Elderflower (for detoxification and mild oestrogenic activity)
- 1-2 slices of fresh Lemon (optional, for added freshness and vitamin C)
- 1 teaspoon raw honey or sweetener

Instructions:
1. Start by boiling about 2 cups of water in a kettle or on the stovetop.
2. Place all of the dried flowers (hibiscus,

chamomile, lavender, red clover, and elderflower) into a tea infuser or tea bag. If you don't have an infuser, you can simply add the herbs directly into the teapot or cup, and strain them after steeping.

3. Pour the hot water over the herbs and let it steep for about 5-7 minutes. The longer it steeps, the more intense the flavour and benefits.

4. Add fresh lemon slices for a refreshing citrus note and a boost of vitamin C. You can also sweeten your tea with a teaspoon of raw honey or your favourite sweetener if desired.

5. If you used loose herbs, strain the tea into your mug. If you used an infuser, simply remove it. Enjoy the fragrant, colourful tea!

Additional Tips:

- Frequency: You can drink this tea 1-2 times a day, especially in the evening to help wind down and prepare for restful sleep.

- Cold Option: This tea can also be chilled for a refreshing iced tea, especially in warm weather. Simply steep as usual,

cool down, and refrigerate.
- If you'd like, you can add a pinch of ginger or cinnamon for   added warmth and digestive support.

Meno Spice Mix

Here's how you might blend these ingredients to create a Menopause Spice Mix:
Ingredients:
- 2 tbsp fennel seeds
- 2 tbsp fenugreek seeds
- 1 tbsp turmeric powder
- 1   tbsp ginger   powder or dried   ginger root powder
- 2 tbsp ground flaxseeds
- 1 tsp cinnamon powder
- 1 tsp cardamom powder
- 1   tsp clove   powder (or a few whole cloves, ground)

Instructions:
1. Grind fennel, fenugreek, flaxseeds, and any whole spices (cloves, cardamom) in a spice grinder or mortar and pestle.
2. Mix all the ground spices and powders in a bowl.
3. Store the blend in an airtight jar away

from heat and light to preserve freshness.

How to Use the Spice Mix:
1. A teaspoon or two can be added to your morning smoothie.
2. Sprinkle it over oatmeal, yogurt, roasted vegetables, or salads.
3. Add a teaspoon to hot water, steep for 5-10 minutes, and enjoy a warming, soothing tea.
4. Use it in curry dishes, soups, or any recipe where you would traditionally use spices like turmeric, ginger, or cinnamon.
5. Combine with honey and warm water for a soothing, hormone-balancing drink

Meno Power Plant Butter

This spread now includes more phytoestrogenic and nutrient-dense ingredients for a hormone-balancing boost.
Ingredients:
- ½ cup ground flaxseeds (lignans for oestrogen support)
- ½

  cup walnuts or almonds (phytoestrogens, omega-3s, and healthy fats)

- 3 tablespoons sesame seeds or tahini (high in lignans)
- 6 Medjool dates, pitted (natural sweetness and magnesium)
- 2 tablespoons dried blueberries or cranberries (antioxidants and phytoestrogens)
- 1 teaspoon cinnamon (blood sugar regulation)
- 1 teaspoon vanilla extract
- 1 tablespoon ground pumpkin seeds (rich in magnesium and zinc)
- 2-4 tablespoons water or almond milk (adjust for consistency)

Instructions:

1. In a food processor, blend flaxseeds, walnuts, sesame seeds, and pumpkin seeds into a coarse powder.
2. Add Medjool dates, dried berries, cinnamon, and vanilla extract. Blend until the mixture starts to clump.
3. Gradually add water or almond milk until the mixture is smooth and spreadable.
4. Store in an airtight jar in the refrigerator for up to 2 weeks.

How to Use:

- Spread on whole-grain bread or rice cakes.
- Add a dollop to oatmeal, yogurt, or smoothies.
- Use as a dip for apple or pear slices.

Meno Tahini-Miso Sauce

Ingredients:
- 3 tablespoons tahini (sesame seeds for lignans)
- 1 tablespoon white miso paste (fermented soy for isoflavones)
- 2 tablespoons fresh lemon juice (antioxidants and vitamin C)
- 1 tablespoon flaxseed oil (omega-3s for hormone balance)
- 1 tablespoon ground sunflower seeds (vitamin E for skin and hair health)
- ½ teaspoon turmeric (anti-inflammatory properties)
- ½ teaspoon grated fresh ginger (supports digestion and reduces inflammation)
- 2 teaspoons chopped fresh parsley or dried parsley (mild phytoestrogen content and antioxidants)

- 1 clove garlic, minced (optional, immune support)
- 2-3 tablespoons warm water (to thin the sauce)

Instructions:
1. Whisk tahini, miso paste, and lemon juice in a small bowl until smooth.
2. Gradually whisk in flaxseed oil, ground sunflower seeds, turmeric, ginger, and parsley.
3. Add minced garlic (if using) and warm water, one tablespoon at a time, until the desired consistency is reached.
4. Store in the refrigerator for up to 1 week.

How to Use:
- Drizzle over roasted or steamed vegetables (like broccoli or asparagus).
- Toss with quinoa, brown rice, or sweet potato slices.
- Use as a spread for sandwiches or a dip for raw vegetables.

Meno Quinoa Salad

- Ingredients:
  - 1 cup cooked quinoa

- o 1 diced cucumber
- o 1 chopped endive
- o 1 teaspoon pumpkin seeds
- o Fresh parsley and lemon juice and ½ teaspoon ground fenugreek

- Instructions:
  - o Toss all ingredients together for a nutrient-packed, oestrogen-supporting meal.

Meno Lentil Soup

- Ingredients:
  - o 1 teaspoon coconut oil
  - o 1 cup cooked lentils
  - o 1 cup vegetable broth
  - o Spices (turmeric, fenugreek, pepper, cumin)
- Instructions:
  - o Simmer lentils in broth, add spices, and serve warm

Meno Rich Smoothie

- Ingredients:
  - o 1 cup soy milk

- 1 tablespoon ground flaxseeds
  - ½ cup pomegranate arils
  - ½ cup fresh/frosen blueberries
  - 1 medium carrot (peeled and chopped)
- Instructions:

Blend all ingredients until smooth. Consume fresh.

Meno Mediterranean Bowl

- Ingredients:
  - 1 cup cooked chickpeas
  - 2 tablespoons tahini
  - ½ cup shredded carrots
  - 1 tablespoon toasted sesame seeds
  - 1 teaspoon fennel seed powder
- Instructions:

Combine all ingredients in a bowl. Serve with a drizzle of olive oil and lemon juice.

Meno Flaxseed & Alfalfa Sprout Salad

- Ingredients:
  - 2 tablespoons ground flaxseeds
  - 1 cup alfalfa sprouts
  - ½ cup shredded carrots

- o 1 tablespoon sesame oil
- o 1 teaspoon apple cider vinegar
- Instructions:
Toss all ingredients together. Serve fresh.

Meno Soy and Veggie Stir-Fry

- Ingredients:
    - o 1 cup cubed tofu (lightly fried or steamed)
    - o 1 cup steamed carrots
    - o ½ cup alfalfa sprouts
    - o 1 tablespoon soy sauce
    - o 1 teaspoon toasted sesame seeds
- Instructions:
Lightly stir-fry tofu and carrots. Top with alfalfa sprouts and sesame seeds.

Meno Breakfast Bowl

- Ingredients:
    - o ½ cup cooked oats
    - o 1 tablespoon ground flaxseeds, pumpkin seed and sunflower seeds
    - o ½ cup blueberries
    - o 1 teaspoon honey/agave
- Instructions: Combine and serve warm.

Sweet Potato & Broccoli Meno Bowl

- Ingredients:
    - 1 medium baked sweet potato
    - 1 cup steamed broccoli
    - 2 tablespoons tahini dressing
- Instructions: Assemble ingredients and drizzle with tahini dressing.

Meno Beet & Parsley Salad

- Ingredients:
    - 1 roasted beet (cubed)
    - 10 g fresh parsley
    - 1 tablespoon olive oil
    - 1 teaspoon lemon juice
- Instructions: Toss all ingredients together.

Soy Yogurt & Berry Parfait

Ingredients:
- 1 cup unsweetened soy yogurt (rich in isoflavones for hormone balance)
- ½ cup fresh or frosen mixed berries (antioxidants and vitamin C)
- 2 tablespoons granola (choose low-sugar,

high-fibre options)

- 1 tablespoon hemp seeds (omega-3s and phytoestrogens)
- 1 teaspoon ground flaxseeds (lignans for hormone balance)
- 1-2 teaspoons stevia or monk fruit sweetener (optional, low-sugar sweetener)
-

Instructions:

1. In a glass or bowl, layer ⅓ of the soy yogurt, followed by a layer of berries, granola, hemp seeds, and flaxseeds.
2. Repeat the layers until all ingredients are used, finishing with berries and a sprinkle of hemp seeds on top.
3. If needed, drizzle a small amount of sweetener over the top.

How to Use:

- Ideal as a light dessert, breakfast, or mid-day snack.
- Store in the refrigerator if not consumed immediately (best eaten fresh).

2-Ingredient Dark Chocolate Avocado Mousse

Ingredients:
- 1 ripe avocado (creamy texture, healthy fats, and phytoestrogens)
- 3 tablespoons melted dark chocolate (70% or higher, rich in antioxidants and low sugar)

Instructions:
1. Scoop the flesh of the avocado into a blender or food processor.
2. Add the melted dark chocolate and blend until smooth and creamy.
3. Optional: Chill for 10–15 minutes before serving for a firmer texture.

How to Use:
- Serve in small bowls, optionally topped with a sprinkle of cocoa nibs or a few fresh berries.

3-Ingredient Chocolate Banana Bites

Ingredients:
- 1 banana (natural sweetness and mild phytoestrogen content)
- 50 g melted dark chocolate (70% or

higher, antioxidant-rich)
- 1 tablespoon crushed nuts (e.g., almonds, walnuts, or hazelnuts for phytoestrogens and healthy fats)

Instructions:
1. Slice the banana into bite-sized pieces.
2. Dip each piece halfway into the melted chocolate.
3. Sprinkle with crushed nuts and place on a parchment-lined tray.
4. Chill in the refrigerator until the chocolate hardens (about 15 minutes)

Bon Appetit!

12 Home-made Recipes for External Use

Before we start, yes, phytoestrogens can cross the skin barrier and get absorbed.

Natural Oestrogenic Gel Recipe

Ingredients:
- 3 teaspoons flaxseeds
- 1 cup boiled water
- 1 tablespoon Red Clover Extract (or dried sage)
- 3 whole cloves
- 1 tablespoon ground Fenugreek
- 2 teaspoons Aloe Vera Gel (fresh or store-bought, if fresh, scrape from the plant)
- 1 teaspoon Jojoba Oil (or Sweet Almond Oil)
- 5-10 drops Clary Sage Essential Oil (or Geranium Essential Oil)

Instructions:
1. Combine the Ingredients:
    - In a clean bowl or jar, add

your flaxseeds
- o Cloves, Sage, Red Clover Extract, Fenugreek Mix well.
- o Add the Soy Isoflavones (if you have them) and stir thoroughly to ensure all the active compounds are well distributed.
- o Add 1 cup of freshly boiled water and allow to sit for 2/3 hours.
- o Sieve gel into a clean glass jar.
- o Add the Jojoba Oil (or Sweet Almond Oil) for added hydration and to help with absorption.
- o Finally, add 5-10 drops of Clary Sage or Geranium Essential Oil. These essential oils provide hormonal balancing benefits and also act as a natural preservative for the gel.

2. Store:
- o Store it in the refrigerator for up to a week to keep it fresh and cool.

To Use:
- Apply a small amount of the gel to your skin, focusing on areas like the inner forearms, lower abdomen, or thighs,

where absorption is often better.
- Gently massage it in, allowing the skin to absorb the gel.
- You can apply this gel once or twice a day, depending on your preference.

This recipe combines natural, easy-to-find ingredients that can help mimic oestrogenic effects while nourishing and moisturizing the skin. Using homemade flaxseed gel means you're not relying on commercial products, and it aligns with your preference for natural, DIY options!

Rosemary Oil Hair Loss

During menopause, hormonal changes, particularly a drop in oestrogen and an increase in dihydrotestosterone (DHT), can lead to hair thinning. Rosemary oil is believed to inhibit the conversion of testosterone to DHT, helping to slow hair loss.

Rosemary oil soothes inflammation in the scalp, which can exacerbate hair loss conditions. The Antioxidant Protection: The compounds in rosemary oil (e.g., carnosic acid) help repair damage in the scalp tissues, promoting healthier follicles. Rosemary Encourages

Some studies have shown rosemary oil to be as effective as minoxidil, a common hair growth treatment, in promoting hair regrowth over a 6-month period, without the side effects.

Rosemary Essential Oil
- Active Compound: Carnosic acid, carnosol, and rosmarinic acid.
- Bioactive Dose:
    - 5-10 drops of rosemary essential oil diluted in 2 tablespoons of carrier oil (e.g., coconut oil or jojoba oil), applied 2-3 times weekly.
    - Alternatively, 4-5 drops added to shampoo for regular use.

DIY Rosemary Floral Oil

Ingredients:
- 1 cup fresh rosemary sprigs (or ½ cup dried rosemary leaves)

- 1 cup carrier oil (e.g., coconut oil, jojoba oil, or sweet almond oil)

Instructions:
1. Prepare the Rosemary:
    - If using fresh rosemary, gently rinse and pat dry to remove any dirt. Ensure the sprigs are completely dry to prevent mold growth in the oil.
2. Infuse the Oil (Method 1: Slow Heat):
    - Place the rosemary sprigs in a small, heat-safe glass jar or saucepan.
    - Pour the carrier oil over the herbs, ensuring they are fully submerged.
    - Heat the jar or saucepan gently using a double boiler or low heat on the stovetop for 2-3 hours. The temperature should not exceed 120°F (50°C) to preserve the beneficial compounds.

Infuse the Oil (Method 2: Sunlight):
    - Place the rosemary and oil mixture in a sterilised glass jar with a tight lid.

- o Let it sit in a sunny windowsill for 2-4 weeks, shaking occasionally to encourage infusion.
3. Strain the Oil:
   - o Once infused, strain the mixture using a fine mesh strainer or cheesecloth and transfer the strained oil into a sterilised glass bottle or jar.
4. Optional Additions:
   - o Add 3-5 drops of rosemary essential oil to boost the potency.
   - o Add a few drops of vitamin E oil to extend shelf life.

How to Use:

- Massage a small amount of the oil into your scalp, focusing on areas of thinning hair.
- Leave it on for 30 minutes to overnight, then rinse with a gentle shampoo.
- Use 2-3 times per week for best results.

Storage:

- Store the oil in a cool, dark place. It will keep for up to 6 months if properly stored.

Meno Moisturiser

Ingredients:
- 2 tbsp shea butter (deeply moisturizing and rich in vitamins A and E)
- 1 tbsp coconut oil (locks in moisture)
- 1 tbsp flaxseed oil (rich in lignans, a potent phytoestrogen)
- 1 tsp evening primrose oil (supports elasticity and combats dryness)
- 3 drops lavender essential oil (soothes skin and adds a calming scent)
- 3 drops geranium essential oil (balances hormones and improves hydration)

Instructions:
1. Melt the shea butter and coconut oil in a double boiler or microwave on low heat.
2. Remove from heat and stir in flaxseed oil and evening primrose oil.
3. Add lavender and geranium essential oils, mixing well.
4. Pour the mixture into a jar and allow it to cool and solidify.
5. Apply morning and night to the face and any areas of dry skin.

Meno Mascara

Ingredients:
- 1/2 tsp activated charcoal (for colour)
- 1/4 tsp bentonite clay (improves lash adherence)
- 1/4 tsp aloe vera gel (hydrates lashes)
- 1/4 tsp flaxseed gel (rich in lignans, nourishes lashes and adds smooth texture)
- 2 drops vitamin E oil (preserves the mixture and strengthens lashes)

Instructions:
1. Warm the aloe vera gel and flaxseed gel together until slightly thickened.
2. Stir in the activated charcoal and bentonite clay to create a smooth, lump-free paste.
3. Add vitamin E oil for preservation and nourishment.
4. Transfer to a clean mascara tube and apply with a mascara wand.

Meno Rouge/Lip Gloss Combo

Ingredients:
- 1 tsp beetroot powder (for colour and added antioxidants)
- 1 tsp arrowroot powder (for smooth application)
- 1/4 tsp flaxseed gel (phytoestrogen-rich base for hydration)
- 1/4 tsp sesame oil (rich in lignans and provides a dewy finish)
- 1/8 tsp cocoa powder (optional, for a warm undertone)

Instructions:
1. Mix beetroot powder and arrowroot powder in a small bowl.
2. Add flaxseed gel and sesame oil, stirring until a creamy consistency forms.
3. Add cocoa powder for a warmer shade, if desired.
4. Store in a small, clean tin or jar.
5. Apply to lips as a gloss or dab lightly on cheeks for a natural flush.

13 Herbals & Nutraceuticals

The following herbs are all commonly used for menopausal symptom relief, such as hot flush/flashes, mood swings, and hormone balance, **but they should always be used with care and ideally under the guidance of a healthcare provider as they can cause side effects.** If you're considering incorporating them into your routine, it is best to ensure there are no contraindications with any existing medications or conditions.

Black Cohosh
- Active Compound: Triterpene glycosides (primarily actein and cimicifugoside).
- Bioactive Dose:
    - Black cohosh root extract: 20-80 mg per day, typically in capsule or tablet form.
    - Tea: 1-2 teaspoons dried root brewed in 1 cup of water, 1-2 times per day.
- Time to See Effects: Typically, 2-4 weeks for symptom relief (e.g., hot flush/flashes, night sweats).

- Preparation/Processing:
  - Best:
    - Use standardised extracts in supplement form (20-80 mg/day).
    - Brewed tea from dried root, though potency may be less than standardised supplements.
  - Avoid:
    - Overuse beyond recommended dosage, as it can lead to digestive upset or liver stress with prolonged high doses.
    - Self-dosing without medical guidance, especially for women with a history of liver disease.

Chaste Tree (Vitex)
- Active Compound: Iridoid glycosides (primarily agnuside and vitexin).
- Bioactive Dose:
  - Vitex extract: 20-40 mg per day, typically in capsule or tablet form.
  - Tea: 1-2 teaspoons dried berries

brewed in 1 cup of water, 1-2 times per day.

- Time to See Effects: 4-6 weeks (may take longer for full effects).
- Preparation/Processing:
  - Best:
    - Standardised extract in capsule form for consistent dosage.
    - Tea for general use, but extract is more potent for hormonal regulation.
  - Avoid:
    - Overuse, as it can interact with certain medications (e.g., birth control, HRT).
    - Long-term use without breaks to avoid affecting the hypothalamic-pituitary-gonadal axis.

Dong Quai (Angelica Sinensis)
- Active Compound: Phytoestrogens (primarily ferulic acid and ligustilide).
- Bioactive Dose:
  - Dong quai extract: 150-300 mg per day.

- o Tea: 1-2 teaspoons dried root brewed in 1 cup of water, 1-2 times per day.
- Time to See Effects: Typically, 2-4 weeks for symptom relief.
- Preparation/Processing:
  - o Best:
    - Use standardised extract for consistent dosages.
    - Tea or powder form for general use.
  - o Avoid:
    - Overuse, as dong quai may increase bleeding risk, especially when combined with blood-thinning medications (e.g., warfarin).
    - Using during pregnancy due to potential uterine-stimulating effects.

Maca Root

- Active Compound: Macamides and macaenes (compounds unique to maca).
- Bioactive Dose:
  - o Maca powder: 1.5-3 grams per day (usually mixed into smoothies or

water).
- o Capsules: 500-1500 mg per day.
- Time to See Effects: Typically, 2-4 weeks for energy, mood, and libido benefits.

- Preparation/Processing:
  - o Best:
    - Use in powder form (organic maca powder) or capsules for consistent daily dosing.
    - Can be added to smoothies, oatmeal, or baked goods.
  - o Avoid:
    - High doses for extended periods, as maca can affect thyroid function in some individuals.
    - Overconsumption, as it may cause mild digestive upset.

Red Clover
- Active Compound: Isoflavones (primarily genistein and daidsein).
- Bioactive Dose:
  - o Red clover extract: 40-80 mg per day.
  - o Tea: 1-2 teaspoons dried flowers

> brewed in 1 cup of water, 1-2 times per day.

- Time to See Effects: Typically, 2-4 weeks.
- Preparation/Processing:
  - Best:
    - Use in supplement form for standardised doses of isoflavones.
    - Tea for general use, but extract is often more effective for symptom relief.
  - Avoid:
    - Overconsumption, especially for women with hormone-sensitive conditions (e.g., breast cancer), as it may increase oestrogen activity.

Wild Yam

- Active Compound: Diosgenin (a saponin)
- Bioactive Dose:
  - Wild yam root: 200-500 mg per day (typically in supplement form or as part of a combination with other herbs).

- o Wild yam cream: Applied topically according to product instructions (typically 1-2 pumps per day).
  - o Wild yam tea: 1 teaspoon dried root brewed in 1 cup of water, 1-2 times per day.
- Time to See Effects: Typically, 4-6 weeks for symptom relief (though this can vary).
- Preparation/Processing:
  - o Best:
    - Use supplements or extracts in capsule/tablet form.
    - Topical creams may be applied directly to the skin for relief from vaginal dryness or skin hydration.
    - Tea can be made with dried root for general use.
  - o Avoid:
    - Overuse or prolonged high-dose supplementation, as there are concerns about long-term safety and the lack of evidence for effectiveness in large doses.

14 Bibliography

Aromates.clouds (2023) Menopause Memoir. KDP publishing. ASIN : B0CNQ6K6L9

Bull ,F.C., Al-Ansari, S.S., Biddle S, et al., (2020). World Health Organization 2020 guidelines on physical activity and sedentary behaviour British Journal of Sports Medicine, 54(24),1451-1462

Chohan, M., & Morrone, J. (2024). Edible Flowers. KPD publishing ISBN: 9798345970911

De Franciscis, P., Colacurci, N., Riemma, G., Conte, A., Pittana, E., Guida, M., & Schiattarella, A. (2019). A nutraceutical approach to menopausal complaints. *Medicina, 55*(9), 544.

Department of Health (2016) Alcohol Guidelines Review—Report From the Guidelines Development Group to the UK Chief Medical Officers.

Ebrahimi, A., Tayebi, N., Fatemeh, A., & Akbarzadeh, M. (2020). Investigation of the role of herbal medicine, acupressure, and acupuncture in the menopausal symptoms: An evidence-based systematic review study. *Journal of family medicine and primary care, 9*(6), 2638-2649.

England, P. H. (2016). The Eatwell Guide. Available at: www.gov.uk/government/publications/the-eatwell-guide

Huntley, A. (2004). Drug-herb interactions with herbal medicines for menopause. *British Menopause Society Journal, 10*(4), 162-165.

Kargozar, R., Azizi, H., & Salari, R. (2017). A review of effective herbal medicines in controlling menopausal symptoms. *Electronic physician, 9*(11), 5826.

Kronenberg, F., & Fugh-Berman, A. (2002). Complementary and alternative medicine for menopausal symptoms: a review of randomised, controlled trials. *Annals of internal medicine, 137*(10), 805-813.

McMain, S., Newman, M. G., Segal, Z. V., & DeRubeis, R. J. (2015). Cognitive behavioral therapy: Current status and future research directions. *Psychotherapy Research, 25*(3), 321–329. https://doi.org/10.1080/10503307.2014.1002440

Mahdavian, M., Najmabadi, K. M., Hosseinzadeh, H., Mirzaeian, S., Aval, S. B., & Esmaeeli, H. (2019). Effect of the mixed herbal medicines extract (Fennel, Chamomile, and Saffron) on menopause syndrome: A randomised controlled clinical trial. *Journal of caring sciences*, *8*(3), 181.

Martin, C. J. H., Watson, R. R., & Preedy, V. R. (Eds.). (2013). *Nutrition and diet in menopause* (p. 469). Humana Press.

Officers, U. C. M. (2019). UK chief medical officers' physical activity guidelines. United Kingdom Department of Health and Social Care, Llwodraeth Cymru Welsh Government, Department of Health Northern Ireland and the Scottish Government.

Opara, E. I., & Chohan, M. (2021). *Culinary Herbs and Spices: A Global Guide*. The Royal Society of Chemistry

Riemann, D., Baglioni, C., Bassetti, C.. . . Spiegelhalder, K. (2017). European guideline for the diagnosis and treatment of insomnia. *Journal of Sleep Research*, *26*(6), 675–700. https://doi.org/10.1111/jsr.12594

Silva TR, Oppermann K, Reis FM, Spritzer PM. Nutrition in Menopausal Women: A Narrative Review. *Nutrients*. 2021; 13(7):2149. https://doi.org/10.3390/nu13072149

My own Recipes:

My own recipes:

My own recipes:

All the best on your menopause journey.

Thank you,

Mags